BEYOND CALORIES

DISCOVER THE REAL CAUSES OF OBESITY AND HOW TO OVERCOME THEM

Steve N. Cone

TABLE OF CONTENTS

INTRODUCTION 4

CHAPTER 1: THE OBESITY TERM 6

CHAPTER 2: THE ODDITIES OF OBESITY 10

CHAPTER 3: UNDERSTANDING THE ROLE OF CALORIES 14

CHAPTER 4: BEYOND CALORIES 21

CHAPTER 5: A NOVEL HOPE 34

FINAL SUMMARY 44

INTRODUCTION

For a very long time, calories have been considered the gold standard for weighing food and assessing how it affects our bodies. This book dares to go beyond the superficial level of calorie counting and asks you to examine the deeper dimensions of your well-being in a world where numbers on a scale and the persistent pursuit of fad diets are idolised.
But as we learn more about the nuances of human physiology and nutrition, we come to understand that health is so much more than just a number. Our bodies are complex systems that are intricately linked and impacted by a multitude of factors that go well beyond the calories we put in and track.

"Beyond Calories," presents a life-changing trip that dispels myths about health and gives you the tools to adopt a holistic approach to wellness.

We set out on a mission to discover the hidden realities about diet, exercise, and lifestyle decisions that have the potential to significantly affect our general well-being in Beyond Calories. This book is not about short cuts or band-aid fixes; rather, its goal is to give you the information and skills necessary to develop long-lasting habits and promote a healthy connection with your body.

With the support of cutting-edge scientific findings and ancient wisdom, the book Beyond Calories provides a thorough road map for overcoming the constraints of conventional health advice. Whether your goals are to reduce extra weight, increase your energy, or develop a stronger feeling of self-awareness, this book will guide you towards a new paradigm of wellness.

CHAPTER 1:

THE OBESITY TERM

Obesity is a condition characterized by excessive body fat that negatively impacts health, has been on the rise in recent years. Various factors, including dietary changes, sedentary lifestyles, genetic predispositions, psychological issues, and environmental influences, contribute to this increase. To effectively address the obesity epidemic, it is crucial to understand the interconnectedness of these factors.

In our current circumstances, many individuals find it increasingly challenging to maintain a healthy diet and engage in sufficient physical activity, thereby contributing to the escalating obesity rates.

People are classified as obese when their body mass index (BMI) is over 30kg/m^2; the range 25 to 30 kg/m^2 is defined as overweight.
Some East Asian countries use lower values to calculate obesity.

NB- Body Mass Index (BMI) is a person's weight divided by the square of the person's height.

For most adults, if your BMI is:
Below 18.5–you're in the underweight range,
18.5 to 24.9–you're in the healthy weight range,
25 to 29.9–you're in the overweight range,
30 to 39.9–you're in the obese range,
40 or above–you're in the severely obese range.

You must use a lower BMI score to determine overweight and obesity if you come from a South Asian, Chinese, other Asian, Middle Eastern, Black African, or African-Caribbean family:

23 to 27.4–you're in the overweight range
27.5 or above–you're in the obese range.

CAUSES OF OBESITY:

A complex problem with numerous causes is obesity.
Extra calories, especially from foods high in fat and sugar, are stored as fat in the body and lead to obesity and overweight.
For some people, genetics may also be the cause of their obesity. The way your body stores fat and uses food is influenced by your genes. Sometimes, underlying medical conditions like hypothyroidism—an underactive thyroid gland—can lead to weight gain. However, if these conditions are adequately treated with medication, weight problems usually do not result from them.

Certain medications, such as steroids and some treatments for high blood pressure, diabetes, or mental health issues, can also increase a person's risk of gaining weight.

Why Is That An Issue?

Obesity can lead to various serious medical conditions, including diabetes and heart disease. It also diminishes our ability to enjoy life to the fullest, as we may experience fatigue, lack of energy, or other health issues.

Obesity is a significant cause of disability and is associated with various diseases and conditions, including cardiovascular disease, type 2 diabetes, obstructive sleep apnea, certain cancers, and osteoarthritis.

HOW OBESITY SPREADS

It is well known that friends can become obese together, but how does this happen?

Social spread of obesity is more likely to occur when friends engage in activities and share surroundings that can lead to weight gain than when they have similar views about what constitutes an acceptable body size. Put another way, shared social norms are probably not as important in the obesity "friend effect" as shared social behaviors, like dining out, and shared environments.

The sharp increase in obesity rates in the US has been the subject of intense investigation by public health officials. The rising statistics are undoubtedly influenced by a number of clear factors, including a sedentary lifestyle and poor eating habits. Nevertheless, the emphasis of these and other explanations is frequently limited to how a person's decisions and actions influence their weight.

CHAPTER 2:

THE ODDITIES OF OBESITY

(The Problems Associated With Obesity And Weight Gain)

Obesity has significant consequences for both the body and mind. Our bodies are interconnected, with weight affecting various aspects of our health. Maintaining a healthy weight is crucial for the optimal functioning of our bones, muscles, brain, heart, and other organs. Excess weight, especially obesity, negatively impacts almost every aspect of our health, from memory and mood to respiratory and reproductive systems.

Obesity increases the risk of several diseases, including diabetes, heart disease, and certain types of cancer. It is a major health concern that affects individuals, society, and healthcare costs. Obesity not only shortens life expectancy and reduces quality of life but also exacerbates mental health issues such as depression and low self-esteem.

Fortunately, losing weight can help mitigate some of the risks associated with obesity. Even losing as little as 5 to 10 percent of body weight can have significant health benefits, regardless of whether an obese individual reaches their "ideal" weight or starts losing weight later in life.

OBESITY AND DIABETES

Type 2 diabetes is heavily influenced by body weight. Studies have shown that individuals with a body mass index (BMI) of 35 or higher are at a significantly increased risk of developing diabetes compared to those with lower BMIs. Even individuals with healthy BMIs can increase their risk of diabetes by gaining weight in adulthood. The association between weight and diabetes is consistent across genders.

Research has also shown that fat cells, particularly those around the abdomen, release hormones and chemicals that fuel inflammation. While inflammation is a natural part of the body's immune response, excessive inflammation can lead to various health issues. Inflammation can affect insulin resistance, fat and carbohydrate metabolism, and ultimately raise blood sugar levels, leading to diabetes and its complications. Several large trials have demonstrated that moderate weight loss can delay or prevent the onset of diabetes in high-risk individuals.

OBESITY AND CARDIOVASCULAR DISEASE

Body weight is directly linked to numerous cardiovascular risk factors. As BMI increases, blood pressure, LDL cholesterol, triglycerides, glucose levels, and inflammation all rise. These changes significantly increase the risk of heart disease, stroke, and cardiovascular death.

OBESITY AND CANCER

The relationship between obesity and cancer is not as straightforward as it is with diabetes and cardiovascular disease, primarily because cancer encompasses a variety of diseases rather than a single condition. However, research has found convincing evidence linking obesity to cancers of the esophagus, pancreas, colon and rectum, breast, endometrium, kidney, and potentially gallbladder. Adult obesity and weight gain have also been associated with various other cancers. Encouragingly, the Nurses' Health Study has shown that losing weight after menopause can significantly reduce postmenopausal cancer risk for overweight women who have never used hormone replacement therapy.

OBESITY AND MORTALITY

Obesity has a negative impact on overall mortality rates, including premature death. However, determining the role of weight in premature mortality is challenging due to systemic issues and confounding factors. BMI under 25 includes both healthy individuals and those who have lost weight due to illness, such as cancer. Smoking further complicates matters, as smokers generally weigh less than nonsmokers. When reverse causation and the adverse effects of smoking are not accounted for, death rates among lean individuals are inflated, while those among overweight and obese individuals are reduced. Correcting for statistical biases has shown a significant increase in obesity-related excess deaths compared to initial estimates. Multiple studies have demonstrated a similar relationship between weight and mortality, with an increased risk of death from any cause, cardiovascular disease, cancer, and other illnesses as BMI increases above certain thresholds.

THE BOTTOM LINE

Corpulence adversely affects pretty much every part of wellbeing, from decreasing future and adding to constant circumstances like diabetes and cardiovascular infection to obstructing sexual capability, breathing, mind-set, and social connections. Corpulence isn't generally a long-lasting condition. Weight reduction can be accomplished through diet, exercise, prescriptions, and even surgery.However, getting in shape is significantly more troublesome than acquiring it. Weight counteraction, starting early on and going on all through one's life, can possibly boundlessly work on individual and general wellbeing, diminish enduring, and save billions of dollars in medical care costs every year.

CHAPTER 3:

UNDERSTANDING THE ROLES OF CALORIES

Scarcely any ideas certainly stand out enough to be noticed in the study of weight the executives and nourishment as calories. The customary view on calories and weight gain has pervaded the public cognizance for a really long time, characterizing our insight about how our bodies use energy. Be that as it may, not every person who lives in such conditions will become large, nor will all hefty individuals have a similar muscle versus fat dissemination or experience similar medical issues.

Nonetheless, as how we might interpret nourishment and the intricacies of human digestion has developed, it has become evident that the customary perspective on calories has limitations. This part dives into the hypothesis of calories, exploring their estimation, computation, and the disadvantages of depending entirely on calorie counting for weight reduction.

WHAT ARE CALORIES?

Calories are a unit of energy that is usually used to work out the energy content of food sources and drinks.

A dietary calorie is deductively characterized as how much intensity energy expected to raise the temperature of one kilogram of water by one degree Celsius.

Calories are expected for your body to work and are utilized to drive three significant cycles:

BMR (Basal Metabolic Rate): This is the quantity of calories expected to keep up with your major requirements, like your cerebrum, kidneys, heart, lungs, and sensory system.

Processing: To process and use the food sources you eat, your body exhausts a specific number of calories. Thermic effect of food (TEF) is one more term for this.

Digestion: To digest and metabolize the foods you eat, your body expends a certain number of calories. Thermic effect of food (TEF) is another term for this.

Physical Activity: This is the number of calories required to fuel your daily tasks and physical activity.

Calorie Intake

Several factors influence how many calories a person should consume per day in order to lose weight effectively. Several of these elements are as follows::

•Desired level of weight loss

•Desired speed of weight loss

•Age of individual

•Sex of individual, etc.

Measuring and Calculating Calories

To fathom the job of calories, you should initially comprehend how they are estimated and determined. Bomb calorimetry, which includes consuming an example of food and estimating the intensity delivered, is the most famous way for working out calories in food. This strategy, in any case, doesn't consider the intricacies of human assimilation and digestion. Thus, food marks and calorie-counting applications every now and again depend on supplement data sets, which decide calorie content utilizing middle qualities.

Calculating calories exhausted through actual work is additionally troublesome. The creation of the body age, orientation, hereditary qualities, and individual metabolic rates all affect how much energy is used during exercise. Conventional equations and movement trackers can give good guesses, yet they don't consider every individual's particular highlights

The Conventional View on Calories and Weight Gain

Calories have been generally perceived as the essential unit of energy with regards to nourishment. As per the customary way of thinking, weight gain or misfortune still up in the air by the equilibrium of calories ingested and calories used. Taking in additional calories than the body consumes brings about weight gain, while consuming less calories brings about weight reduction. This improved on perspective has filled in as the establishment for the vast majority famous eating regimens and weight reduction strategies.

Essentially confining your caloric admission can influence your digestion and prompt you to lose bulk.

This can make it challenging to keep up with weight reduction long haul, and confining your calorie consumption an excess of can prompt weakness.

Keeping up with this calorie limitation for a really long time can prompt healthful lacks.

Knowing the viability of a diet is preposterous all of the time.

Confining caloric admission also seriously can influence richness, particularly in ladies.

Further exploration is expected to decide the impacts of calorie limitation in men.

Confining your calorie admission can disturb your chemical levels, debilitating your bones and expanding your gamble of cracks.

Calorie limitation can debilitate the invulnerable framework, particularly when joined with arduous actual work.

<u>Limitations of Using Calorie Counting as The Sole Approach to Weight Management</u>

1. Nutrient Quality: Calorie counting centers dominatingly around amount, dismissing the nature of the food ate. This approach neglects to think about the healthy benefit, like nutrients, minerals, and phytochemicals present in various food varieties. Subsequently, people who exclusively center around meeting their calorie target might wind up with an

eating regimen coming up short on fundamental supplements, which can prompt inadequacies and medical problems.

2. Individual Contrast: Calorie needs change among people because of elements like digestion, body structure, age, sex, and movement level. A "one-size-fits-all" way to deal with calorie counting disregards these singular distinctions. Two individuals with a similar calorie admission might encounter various results as far as weight reduction or gain because of varieties in their metabolic rates.

3. Accuracy of Calorie Estimations: Calorie counts listed on food labels or in calorie-counting apps are often approximations that may not be entirely accurate. There can be variations in nutrient composition due to factors like cooking methods, food processing, and individual food variations. Moreover, accurately measuring portion sizes can be challenging, leading to inaccuracies in calorie calculations.

4. Psychological Impact: Calorie counting can become obsessive and lead to an unhealthy relationship with food. Constantly tracking and restricting calories may cause stress, anxiety, and an unhealthy preoccupation with food. It can contribute to disordered eating patterns, such as orthorexia (obsession with healthy eating) or anorexia nervosa.

5. Ignoring Satiety and Hunger Cues: Focusing solely on calorie numbers can lead to ignoring important hunger and satiety cues from the body. Some foods may be more satiating than others, even if they have the same calorie content. Ignoring these cues can lead to unsatisfying meals, increased cravings, and potential overeating or undereating.

6. Impact on Social Life and Eating Out: Calorie counting can make social situations challenging. It may restrict individuals

from enjoying meals at restaurants or social events, causing feelings of isolation and anxiety. The emphasis on calorie counting can interfere with the enjoyment of food and the social aspects of eating.

7. Long-Term Sustainability: Calorie counting is often seen as a short-term solution for weight loss rather than a sustainable lifestyle change. It can be tedious and time-consuming to track every calorie consumed. Once individuals achieve their weight goals, they may struggle to maintain the habit of counting calories in the long run, potentially leading to weight regain.

8. Metabolic Adaptation: The body has a remarkable ability to adapt to changes in calorie intake. When calorie intake is reduced, the body may respond by slowing down metabolism to conserve energy, making weight loss more difficult. This metabolic adaptation can undermine the effectiveness of calorie counting as a weight management strategy

9. Limited Focus on Overall Health: Weight management is not solely about calories. It involves overall health, including exercise, sleep, stress management, and emotional well-being. Relying solely on calorie counting neglects these important aspects of a healthy lifestyle, which can impact weight management and overall well-being.

THE BOTTOM LINE

Tolerance is fundamental for long haul weight decrease. It's ideal to stay away from eats less that expect you to limit your calorie admission harshly.

While calories truly do assume a part in weight the board, it is vital to comprehend the disadvantages and requirements of utilizing calorie considering the main methodology. Some are upheld by proof, are protected, and productive, while others are not. Numerous wellbeing experts, dietitians, and nutritionists concur that coordinating a solid, weight reduction diet with customary actual work yields the best results, especially after some time.

Knowing the complexities of sustenance, varieties among individuals, and the significance of generally speaking wellbeing is basic for compelling and long haul weight decrease. An amicable methodology that considers supplement quality, individual necessities, and all encompassing wellbeing is fundamental for long haul weight control a positive outcome. We can lay out a more itemized and customized way to deal with solid living by growing our figuring out past the customary reasoning of calories.

CHAPTER 4:

BEYOND CALORIES

<u>Introduction</u>

Obesity is a many-sided condition that outcomes from various factors other than the admission of calories. In this part, we will take a gander at the numerous features of stoutness, including the hereditary, hormonal, metabolic, and ecological variables which adds to its headway. Understanding the genuine reasons for weight permits us to expose normal fantasies and foster a more definite way to deal with counteraction and treatment.

GENETIC FACTORS

Obesity can be influenced by genetics, but it is important to note that it is not the only factor. The intricate connection between genetic factors and environmental influences such as diet and lifestyle adds to the advancement of obesity.

Here Are A Few Ways In Which Genetics Can Influence Obesity:

1. GENETIC PREDISPOSITION: Certain individuals have a hereditary inclination to acquire pounds all the more effectively or have more slow metabolic rate. Certain qualities can impact hunger guidelines, digestion, as well as fat safeguarding and dispersion in the body. Varieties in these qualities can incline certain individuals toward weight gain and corpulence more than others.

2. LEPTIN PATHWAY: Leptin is a hormone that controls hunger and energy balance. Mutations or variations in genes involved in the leptin pathway can disrupt normal signaling, resulting in increased appetite and reduced energy consumption, which may give rise to obesity.

3. FAT STORAGE AND METABOLISM: Fat storage and metabolism genes may contribute to an individual's susceptibility to obesity. Some people, for instance, may have genes that encourage the storage of excess calories as fat, making it difficult for them to sustain a healthy weight.

4. GUT MICROBIOTA: Qualities related with fat capacity and digestion might add to a singular's weakness to weight. Certain individuals, for instance, may have qualities that advance gathering of fat, making it challenging for them to keep an optimal weight.

5. GENE-ENVIRONMENT INTERACTION: While genetics may raise one's possibility of obesity, it is also important to recognise that external influences play a role. Obesity risk is increased when poor

dietary habits, sedentary lifestyles, limited access to nutritious foods, and other environmental factors cooperate with a person's genetic makeup.

It is essential to note that having a genetic predisposition to overweight does not automatically mean that a person will eventually become obese. Physical activity, for example, can still have a major impact on weight management.

HORMONAL IMBALANCES

Hormones that regulate appetite, metabolism, and fat storage include leptin, ghrelin, insulin, and cortisol. These hormone imbalances can impair the body's ability to maintain a healthy weight. hormonal deficiencies and weight gain can be exacerbated by conditions such as polycystic ovary syndrome (PCOS) and hypothyroidism.

INSULIN

Insulin is a hormone which controls blood sugar (glucose) levels. It is made by the beta cells of the pancreatic islets of Langerhans.

Its primary function is to allow glucose into cells for use as fuel. Insulin manages blood sugar levels during digestion to supply energy to organs and tissues. It causes fat cells to absorb excess glucose for storage and prevents stored fat from being released for energy. When insulin becomes resistant, its signals to absorb glucose are not properly adhered to, which causes issues

When the level of blood glucose falls, secretion of insulin stops and the liver releases glucose into the blood.

A healthy adult's pancreas contains roughly 200 units of insulin, and the typical regular secretion of insulin into transportation ranges from 30 to 50 units.

Several factors stimulate insulin secretion, but the percentage of glucose in arterial (oxygenated) blood that perfuses the islets is by far the most relevant. When blood glucose levels rise (for example, after a meal), beta cells take up and metabolize a large amount of glucose, and insulin secretion rises. Conversely, as blood glucose concentrations fall, so does insulin secretion; however, small amounts of insulin are secreted even during fasting.

Certain amino acids, fatty acids, keto acids (products of fatty acid oxidation), and several hormones secreted by the gastrointestinal tract may also stimulate release of insulin. Insulin secretion is hampered by somatostatin and sympathetic nervous system activation (the branch of the autonomic nervous system accountable for the fight-or-flight response).

Insulin Problems

In certain individuals, the safe framework goes after the islets, making them quit delivering insulin or to create lacking sums. At the point when this occurs, blood glucose stays in the blood and cells can't retain it to change over the sugars into energy. This is the beginning of type 1 diabetes, and an individual with this sort of diabetes will require continuous infusions of insulin to get by.

In certain individuals, especially the people who are overweight, corpulent, or idle, insulin is ineffectual in conveying glucose into cells and can't do its capabilities. Insulin opposition alludes to the failure of insulin to apply its impact on tissues. Type 2 diabetes is created when the islets can't deliver sufficient insulin to defeat the condition.

Scientists in the clinical field have found that cutting calories from food, working out, keeping a sound, adjusted diet, and getting satisfactory rest can all guide in weight reduction. An individual may once in a while track down that weight reduction medical procedure, for example, bariatric medical procedure, is valuable.

Unnecessary weight reduction can sometimes be unsafe to one's wellbeing. Please, an individual ought to counsel a specialist prior to making dietary or exercise changes.

The Impacts of Insulin Resistance

Genetics, obesity, and a sedentary lifestyle can all increase insulin resistance through unclear mechanisms. Instead of being assimilated, blood sugar levels rise when cells do not react to insulin as they should. The pancreas strains to make more insulin, which eventually impairs the organ's ability to operate properly. Reduced signals to store fat are also associated with lower insulin sensitivity. As a result, energy excess stays in the system and encourages additional fat storage.

THE ROLE OF LEPTIN

The chemical leptin, which was first found during the 1990s, is a pivotal flagging framework that interfaces the nerve center's control of craving and fat stores. Made in fat cells, it cautions the cerebrum when put away energy is sufficient to smother hunger. The cerebrum doesn't get the "full" message in insulin-safe states due to leptin obstruction, which makes signals pointless even in instances of high muscle versus fat. In this manner, even in circumstances where stores are overloaded, craving is as yet prompted.

Clinical And Population Impact

Longitudinal studies have shown that these interruptions raise an individual's risk of obesity, diabetes, cardiovascular disease, and metabolic syndrome (Megan 2015). Parallel spikes are seen in populations whose nutrition shifts to high-fat/high-sugar diets as their metabolic health deteriorates. Clinical research suggests that lifestyle modifications emphasizing activity, stress reduction, and balanced whole foods are the most successful in enhancing sensitivity.

CORTISOL

A characteristic pressure chemical, it is liable for directing your digestion, so it's vital to keep normal wellbeing rules to bring it down. From carving out opportunities for unwinding to working on your eating regimen and exercise, you can guarantee that you control your cortisol and not the opposite way around.

What Is Cortisol?

Cortisol is a chemical normally delivered by your body. Made by the adrenal organs situated on your kidneys, cortisol is delivered when you're under pressure. This sends your body into survival mode, briefly stopping standard physical processes and easing back your digestion. While this chemical is vital for endurance, it can become unsafe in abundance sums.

How Cortisol Can Lead to Weight Gain

Cortisol invigorates your fat and sugar digestion, making a flood of energy in your body. While this cycle is fundamental for endurance circumstances, it likewise expands your hunger. Also, raised cortisol levels can cause desires for sweet, greasy and pungent food varieties. This implies you're bound to enjoy french fries and a milkshake rather than you are an even feast.

An overabundance of cortisol likewise can lead your body to create less testosterone. This might cause a lessening in bulk, as well as delayed down the number of calories your body consumes.

METABOLIC CONSIDERATIONS

Digestion or metabolic rate is characterized as the series of compound responses in a living organic entity that make and separate energy essential forever. All the more essentially, it's the rate at which your body consumes energy or consumes calories.

Our bodies burn calories in several ways:
1. Through the energy required to keep the body functioning at rest; this is known as your Basal Metabolic Rate (BMR). Your BMR is partly determined by the genes you inherit.
2. Through everyday activities
3. Through exercise

Absorption is essential for the inherited and for the most part past one's compass. Changing it includes amazing conversation. Certain people are basically lucky. They obtained characteristics that advance a faster processing and can eat more than others without gaining weight. Others are not too lucky and end up with a failure to consume calories.

One technique for considering processing is to see your body as an engine that is consistently running. While you're holding on or snoozing, you're engine is sitting like a vehicle at a stop light. A particular proportion of energy is being seared just to keep the engine running. Clearly, for individuals, the fuel source isn't gas. It's the calories found in food sources we eat and rewards we drink, energy that may be used right away or taken care of (especially as fat) for use later.

How quick your body's "motor" runs all things considered, over the long run, decides the number of calories you that consume. In the event that your digestion is "high" (or quick), you will consume more calories very still and during action. An elevated ability to burn calories implies you'll have to take in additional calories to keep up with your weight. That is one justification for why certain individuals can eat more than others without putting on weight. An individual with a "low" (or inability to burn calories) will consume less calories very still and during movement and subsequently needs to eat less to try not to become overweight.

How Does Metabolism Affect Weight?

Numerous people shortcoming metabolic issues for weight fights. However, your assimilation ordinarily guides itself to resolve your body's issues. It's occasional the justification for weight gain or mishap. When in doubt, any person who consumes a more prominent number of calories than they take in will typically shed pounds.

Generally speaking, than lean people during most activities, partially since it requires more work to move around. Nevertheless, they will commonly be more fixed, which makes it harder to discard muscle to fat proportion.

For most of us, changes in weight over a long period are fundamentally impacted by calories in and calories out.

Our bodies are made to store additional energy in fat cells, paying little mind to how rapidly or gradually you consume it off. You will in this manner put on weight assuming that your body utilizes more calories (or "admission") from food and drink than it does (or "yield"). Alternately, you will get more fit in the event that you devour less calories through food and drinks than you consume off during ordinary exercises (like activity, rest, and rest). Moreover, our bodies are wired to decipher a lack of food as starvation. Our BMR dials back thus, consuming less calories over the long run. That is one reason getting more fit is normally hard.

Various speculations exist to get a handle on what controls how much food a singular eats, when they feel full and why they eat past the explanation for feeling full. These components in like manner expect a section in choosing one's conclusive weight. One speculation is that all of us has a set point — a heap at which the body is "euphoric." If you get more fit, you'll feel hungry until you return to your set point weight. That may be another clarification losing excess weight is so troublesome. However, how that permanently set up not set and whether there truly is such a part stay problematic.

Concerning weight, processing is huge and has a genetic part. Whether you can change your metabolic rate, in any case, includes broad conversation. Clearly, you can change how you balance the calories you take in against the calories you consume development, which can change your weight.

THE ROLE OF ENVIRONMENTAL FACTORS, STRESS, OTHER LIFESTYLE FACTORS, AND SEDENTARY HABITS

<u>Stress And Emotional Factors</u>: Constant pressure can add to weight gain and stoutness. Stress sets off the arrival of cortisol, which can increment craving and advance fat stockpiling, especially around the midsection. Stress can fundamentally influence your capacity to keep a solid weight. It can likewise keep you from getting in shape. Whether it's the consequence of elevated degrees of the pressure chemical cortisol, unfortunate pressure prompted ways of behaving, or a mix of the two, the connection among stress and weight gain is glaring. Taking care of

oneself systems like care, journaling, and exercise can assist you with battling pressure and the undesirable impact it can have on your dietary patterns.

Whether or not overabundance measures of cortisol can prompt weight gain is basically equivalent to inquiring as to whether an excess of stress can make you put on undesirable pounds. The response in the two cases is yes.

Close to home variables, like involving food as a survival technique or profound eating, can likewise add to weight gain.

Lifestyle Choices: Obesity is largely caused by sedentary lifestyle choices and inactivity. The increased screen time, desk jobs, and decreased physical activity of modern ways of life have resulted in a decrease in overall energy expenditure. Maintaining an active lifestyle and frequent physical activity are essential for managing weight.

Food Environment: The accessibility and openness of calorie-thick, handled food varieties high in sugar, unfortunate fats, and added substances add to gorging and weight gain. The obesogenic climate, with its overflow of cheap food outlets, huge piece sizes, and food showcasing, settles on it trying to pursue solid choices.

Debunking Common Misconceptions About Causes Of Obesity

"Obesity is solely caused by overeating": The accessibility and openness of calorie-thick, handled food varieties high in sugar, unfortunate fats, and added substances add to gorging and weight gain. The obesogenic climate, with its overflow of inexpensive food outlets, huge part sizes, and food advertising, pursues it trying to settle on solid choices.

"Lack of willpower or laziness causes obesity": It takes more than just resolve or laziness to be obese. It is an intricate interaction of many variables, and those who are obese frequently deal with serious issues relating to metabolism, hormones, heredity, and the external factors.

"All obese individuals have unhealthy eating habits": Being obese requires more than just willpower or sloth. Obesity is often associated with serious problems related to metabolism, hormones, heredity, and environmental variables, all of which interact in a complex way.

Conclusion:

Establishing successful safeguards and curative plans requires an understanding of the real causes of obesity. Through a comprehensive examination of genetic, hormonal, and environmental factors in addition to calorie intake, we can more effectively tackle the multifaceted nature of obesity and advance comprehensive approaches to weight control. By busting myths about obesity, we can gain a more sensitive and in-depth knowledge of the disease, which will lead to better outcomes and a healthier society both now and in the future.

CHAPTER 5:

A NOVEL HOPE

(The Solution Beyond Calorie Counting)

Going with the choice to address your weight is a significant initial move toward rolling out an improvement. Many face a significantly harder choice concluding which strategy they will pick to shed pounds. You might hear individuals discuss picking a "treatment" for their corpulence. This essentially implies concluding which weight reduction technique is appropriate for you.

There are many projects and decisions while checking out weight reduction choices. Every treatment varies from one individual to another, as there is nobody treatment for corpulence. As a purchaser, it is difficult to realize which projects will turn out best for you. As usual, you ought to work with your medical care proficient and examine this large number of choices prior to pursuing a therapy decision. A medical care supplier can best analyze your weight issue and give you the choices as indicated by your wellbeing and way of life. It means quite a bit to work with your Medical care Supplier in this excursion.

WHAT TO EAT AND WHEN TO EAT

Although there may not be a "cure" for obesity, following a healthy eating regimen can help control weight and improve general health. The following are some broad recommendations for controlling weight regarding what to eat as well as when to eat:

1. Focus on a balanced diet: Make sure your meals contain a range of foods that are rich in nutrients. Fruits, vegetables, whole grains, lean meats (like chicken, fish, and legumes), and nutritious fats (found in foods like avocados, nuts, and olive oil) are usually included in this. Make an effort to prepare meals that are well-balanced and contain a healthy combination of micronutrients (minerals and vitamins) and macronutrients (proteins, fats, and carbohydrates).

2. Portion control: Take note of serving sizes to prevent overindulging. To help you manage the amount you eat, use smaller dishes and bowls and pay attention to your body's signals of hunger and fullness. Savour your food and eat slowly to give your body enough time to tell when it is full. When you chew your food, try to count on.

3. Regular meals and snacks: Have three well-balanced meals per day and, if necessary, one or two healthy snacks between meals to develop regular dietary patterns. This can lessen the chance of overeating and stop excessive hunger. However, based on personal desires and requirements, the precise frequency and timing of meals can change.

4. Mindful eating: By being completely in the moment throughout a meal, observing your body's messages of fullness and hunger, and appreciating the flavours and textures of your food, you can practise eating with consciousness. Steer clear of any distractions like screens and juggling different tasks during meals as these can result in mindless overindulgence.

5. Limit processed and sugary foods: Limit the utilization of exceptionally handled food varieties, which are much of the time high in added sugars, undesirable fats, and calories. These food varieties will generally be less filling and can add to weight gain. Choose entire, natural food varieties however much as could be expected.

6. Stay hydrated: Drink a lot of water over the course of the day. In some cases, thirst can be confused with hunger, prompting superfluous eating. Drinking water before feasts can likewise assist you with feeling more full and lessen the probability of gorging.

7. **Seek professional guidance:** Consider speaking with a registered dietitian or other medical professional if you're having trouble controlling your weight or becoming obese. They can offer tailored guidance and assistance according to your particular requirements, state of health, and objectives.

Recall that reaching and maintaining a healthy weight is a gradual process that calls for a variety of lifestyle adjustments, including stress management, regular exercise, healthy eating, and enough sleep. Developing long-term habits that support overall wellness and health is more essential than concentrating on dietary restrictions or short fixes.

Focusing On Whole, Minimally Processed Foods As Much As Possible. This Includes:

- Fish, poultry, and legumes are examples of lean proteins. For satiety, try to limit your meal portions to 3–4 ounces.

- Complex carbohydrates found in starchy vegetables, brown rice, quinoa, and oats. They keep blood sugar levels stable, and fiber keeps you full.
- Vegetables with no starch like peppers, tomatoes, and salad greens that are high in volume but low in calories. Place half of these on your plate.
- Nuts and seeds, avocado, olive oil, and other healthy fats in small quantities. add flavor without adding too many calories.
- Steer clear of liquid calories from drinks like soda, juice, and sweetened coffee as they are high in calories but low in nutrients. Best drinks are water and herbal tea.

As For Timing, It's Ideal To:

- In order to increase metabolism and avoid overindulging later, eat breakfast within an hour of waking up. Fruit, eggs, and oats are all excellent choices.
- For steady energy, eat small meals or snacks every three to four hours that include protein and fiber. Fruit, Greek yogurt, and jerky are portable options.
- For optimal sleep performance, avoid eating two to three hours before bed and allow time for digestion. Save your heaviest meal for an early dinner or lunch.

Pay attention to fullness cues, consume lots of water, and concentrate on satisfying whole foods. Hormone balance gradually becomes better, cravings subside, and a positive, fulfilling interaction with food arises on its own. Remember, Rome wasn't built in a day, so practice self-compassion and patience!

KEEPING PROTEINS CONSUMPTION MODERATE

Modest intake of protein is key to the long-term success of lifestyle modifications aimed at curing obesity and maintaining an appropriate weight. Protein increases metabolism and fills you up, but eating too much of it can be harmful. To lose pounds at a safe, sustainable rate, it is advised to consume 0.5 - 1 grammes of protein per pound of target weight each day.

Spreading admission uniformly over the course of the day in your dinners and snacks is ideal. Great sources incorporate fish, chicken, eggs, nuts, seeds, Greek yogurt and vegetables. At every dinner, protein ought to make up something like 25-30% of what's on your plate. The rest can be loaded up with complex carbs like entire grains, bland vegetables and beans/lentils to give consistent energy while keeping you feeling full.

Be aware of part estimates as well - 3-4 ounces for each dinner is normally adequate. Additionally pay attention to your completion signals so you don't inadvertently go over your protein needs. Overconsumption has been connected to stomach related issues as well as disturbed digestion down the line which can attack weight reduction endeavors. With a decent methodology, moderate protein consumption upholds fat misfortune without negative secondary effects.

BARIATRIC SURGERY

The term "Bariatric Surgery" describes a range of surgical weight reduction techniques used to treat extreme obesity. The three most popular procedures are gastric banding, sleeve gastrectomy, and bypass. These procedures mechanically limit food intake or decrease stomach capacity. Hormone levels and nutritional absorption are abnormally affected by bypassing or cutting off portions of the stomach and/or intestines. For those who qualify, this causes feelings of fullness on less food, resulting in substantial and frequently long-lasting weight loss. For those who are unable to overcome obesity and associated health problems with non-surgical methods alone, bariatric surgery offers an efficient metabolic and anatomical solution.

Below Are Some Key Points On How Bariatric Surgery may help Cure Obesity:

Only those with a body mass index (BMI) of 40 or higher (extreme obesity) or 35–39.9 (severe obesity) plus a medical condition related to obesity, such as diabetes or high blood pressure, are candidates for bariatric processes, such as gastric banding, sleeve gastrectomy, and bypasses.

The way the abdominal surgeries function is that the abdomen is either made smaller (sleeve and band) or reorganized so that the body is able to absorb a certain amount of food at a time (gastric bypass). This reduces hunger and creates the desire of fullness.

On average, patients can expect to lose 50-75% of their excess body weight within 1-2 years after a bariatric operation. However, lifestyle changes are still needed to keep the weight off long-term.

Medical procedure conveys gambles like contamination, spills, blood clumps and nutrient/mineral inadequacies. Broad assessment previously and deep rooted checking after is expected by a doctor. Not every person is an up-and-comer.

Reduction of stoutness related conditions is normal, with diabetes and hypertension for the most part settling quicker than different issues.

For those gathering clinical edges, bariatric medical procedures ought to be viewed as a significant clinical apparatus to treat corpulence when more moderate measures alone have fizzled. Be that as it may, it's anything but an independent arrangement without an integral way of life.

INTERMITTENT FASTING GUIDELINES

Intermittent fasting includes times altogether or to some degree keeping away from eating. There are numerous techniques for discontinuous fasting that shift in the quantity of quick days and the calorie recompenses.

A few investigations recommend that this approach to eating might offer advantages like fat misfortune, work on nature of wellbeing, and life span. Defenders guarantee that a discontinuous fasting program is more straightforward to keep up with than customary, calorie-controlled eats less.

An Intermittent fasting design depends on a set timetable and doesn't follow arbitrary times. All things considered, every individual's insight of discontinuous fasting is individual, and various styles will suit various individuals.

In this part, we examine the famous sorts of irregular fasting and give tips on keeping up with this kind of diet.

1. Fast For 12 Hours A Day

This diet has very easy rules. A person must choose and follow a daily 12-hour window for fasting.

Some researchers claim that if a person fasts for 10 to 16 hours, their body may convert fat reserves into energy and release ketones into the bloodstream. Losing weight ought to be encouraged by this.

For newcomers, this kind of intermittent fasting plan might be a good choice. This is simply because the person is capable of eating the same amount of calories every day, the fasting window is relatively small, and the majority of the fasting takes place during sleep.

The easiest way to do the 12-hour fast is to include the period of sleep in the fasting window.

For example, a person could choose to fast between 7 p.m. and 7 a.m. They would need to finish their dinner before 7 p.m. and wait until 7 a.m. to eat breakfast but would be asleep for much of the time in between.

2. **Fasting for 16 hours**

Fasting for 16 hours a day, leaving an eating window of 8 hours, is called the 16:8 method or the Leangains diet.

During the 16:8 diet, males fast for 16 hours each day, and females fast for 14 hours. This type of intermittent fast may be helpful for someone who has already tried the 12-hour fast but did not see any benefits.

On this fast, people usually finish their evening meal by 8 p.m. and then skip breakfast the next day, not eating again until noon.

A study on mice on a high fat diet found that limiting the feeding window to 8 hours protected them from obesity, inflammation, diabetes, and liver disease, even when they ate the same total number of calories as mice that ate whenever they wished.

3. Fasting for 2 days a week

People following the 5:2 diet eat standard amounts of healthful food for 5 days and reduce calorie intake on the other 2 days.

During the 2 fasting days, males generally consume 600 calories and females 500 calories.

Typically, people separate their fasting days in the week. For example, they may fast on a Monday and Thursday and eat regularly on the other days. There should be at least 1 non-fasting day between fasting days.

There is limited research on the 5:2 diet, which is also known as the Fast diet. A study involving 107 overweight or obese women found that restricting calories twice weekly and continuous calorie restriction both led to similar weight loss.

The study also found that this diet reduced insulin levels and improved insulin sensitivity among participants.

A small-scale study looked at the effects of this fasting style in 23 overweight women. Over the course of one menstrual cycle, the women lost 4.8% of their body weight and 8.0% of their total body fat. However, these measurements returned to usual for most of the women after 5 days of typical eating.

4. Alternate day fasting

There are several variations of the alternate day fasting plan, which involves fasting every other day.

For some people, alternate day fasting means a complete avoidance of solid foods on fasting days, while other people allow up to 500 calories. On feeding days, people often choose to eat as much as they want.

One study reports that alternate day fasting is effective for weight loss and heart health in healthy and overweight adults. The researchers found that the 32 participants lost an average of 5.2 kilograms (kg), or just over 11 pounds (lb), over a 12-week period.

Alternate day fasting is an extreme form of intermittent fasting, and it may not be suitable for beginners or those with certain medical conditions. It may also be difficult to maintain this type of fasting in the long term.

5. **A weekly 24-hour fast**

Fasting completely for 1 or 2 days a week, known as the Eat-Stop-Eat diet, involves eating no food for 24 hours at a time. Many people fast from breakfast to breakfast or lunch to lunch.

People on this diet plan can have water, tea, and other calorie-free drinks during the fasting period.

People should return to regular eating patterns on non-fasting days. Eating in this manner reduces a person's total calorie intake but does not limit the specific foods the individual consumes.

A 24-hour fast can be challenging, and it may cause fatigue, headaches, or irritability. Many people find these effects become less extreme over time as the body adjusts to this new eating pattern.

People may benefit from trying a 12-hour or 16-hour fast before transitioning to the 24-hour fast.

Tips For Maintaining Intermittent Fasting.

It can be challenging to stick to an intermittent fasting program.

The following tips may help you stay on track and maximize the benefits of intermittent fasting:

1. Staying hydrated. Drink lots of water and calorie-free drinks, such as herbal teas, throughout the day. This can help ensure you get enough electrolytes, sodium, and potassium chloride.
2. Avoiding thinking about food. Plan plenty of distractions on fasting days to avoid thinking about food, such as catching up on paperwork or going to see a movie.
3. Resting and relaxing. Avoid strenuous activities on fasting days, although light exercise such as yoga may be beneficial.
4. Making every calorie count. If the chosen plan allows some calories during fasting periods, select nutrient-dense foods that are rich in protein, fiber, and healthful fats. Examples include beans, lentils, eggs, fish, nuts, avocado, and unprocessed meats.
5. Eating high-volume foods. Select filling yet low calorie foods, which include popcorn, raw vegetables, and fruits with high water content, such as grapes and melon.
6. Increasing the taste without the calories. Season meals generously with garlic, herbs, spices, or vinegar. These foods are extremely low in calories yet are full of flavor, which may help to reduce feelings of hunger.
7. Choosing nutrient-dense foods after the fasting period. Eating foods that are high in fiber, vitamins, minerals, and other nutrients helps to keep blood sugar levels steady and prevent nutrient deficiencies.

A **balanced diet** will also contribute to weight loss and overall health. For the best results, it is essential to eat a healthy and balanced diet on non-fasting days. If necessary, a person can seek professional help to personalize an intermittent fasting plan and avoid pitfalls.

People should reach out to a registered dietitian to help them choose the best intermittent fasting plan that fits their lifestyle.

FINAL SUMMARY

In the developed world, obesity is becoming more prevalent and is a public health concern. The issue is that for decades, just-so tales have led us down the garden path, suggesting that cutting out fat from food and losing weight quickly are the solutions. Actually, insulin levels and genetics play a major role in obesity. The actual cause of insulin resistance is not fat per say, but rather the incorrect kind of fat, such as highly refined carbohydrates and sugars, and modified trans fats. Reduce those, and your risk of obesity and associated health problems will be much lower.

We go beyond certain fallacies and misconceptions about obesity that only consider calories and willpower in this educational guide. In this book, the author delves into scientific study to reveal the real physiological and environmental factors contributing to our growing waistlines in the contemporary world. You will discover how our natural systems for regulating our weight are being disrupted at the genetic level by metabolic reactions, long-term stress, and physical inactivity.

However, the book 'Beyond Calories' does not stop with stating challenges and problems; it also offers numerous helpful, lasting remedies that are supported by clinical studies and research. Readers will learn about new ways of life and dietary strategies that restore balance and resilience through nutrition, physical activeness, relaxation, and self-care habits.

This transformative guide, complete with dietary guides, clinical recommendations, and practical tips, empowers readers to reclaim control over their bodies by addressing obesity's fundamental root causes through nutrition and a healthy lifestyle. There are no shortcuts or short-term solutions here, only science-based insights and whole-body tools to support lifelong health goals from within and out.